LIVING WITH
OVARIAN CANCER

The Ultimate Guide To Advance
Approach For Treatment, Diagnosis,
Chemotherapy And Recovery

Dr.Beverly C. Morton

TABLE OF CONTENTS

INTRODUCTION

In a quaint little town nestled amidst rolling hills and lush green landscapes, lived a woman named Khloe. She was a radiant soul, known for her infectious laughter and boundless zest for life. Her days were filled with love, joy, and an unwavering passion for gardening, where she tended to her blooming flowers with meticulous care.

One summer's morning, as the sun painted the sky with hues of gold, Khloe woke up feeling slightly off-kilter. A persistent ache in her abdomen had been bothering her for a few weeks, but she attributed it to the wear and tear of her gardening endeavors. However, this time, the pain was more pronounced and accompanied by an inexplicable fatigue that left her drained and weary.

Concerned, Khloe decided to consult her trusted family physician, Dr. Andrews. As she sat in the cozy waiting room of the quaint clinic, her heart raced with a mix of anticipation and trepidation. The sight of the familiar faces around her, people whose children she had watched grow up, brought a fleeting comfort amidst the uncertainty.

Finally, it was her turn to see the doctor. Dr. Andrews, a compassionate man with kind eyes, listened attentively as Khloe described her symptoms. He asked her a series of questions and performed a thorough examination. After a brief pause, he delivered the news that would forever change Khloe's life.

"Khloe," he said gently, "I want you to know that I am here for you every step of the way. But I have to be honest; the tests indicate that you have ovarian cancer."

Time seemed to stand still as the words reverberated in the room. For Khloe, it felt as if the world had come crashing down around her. The future, once filled with dreams and aspirations, now seemed uncertain and dark.

Yet, amidst the initial shock and fear, Khloe's spirit refused to be defeated. She was determined to fight this battle with all her might, drawing strength from the love of her family and friends who rallied around her, offering unwavering support. Her husband, John, held her hand tightly, assuring her that they were in this together, come what may.

With Dr. Andrews by her side, Khloe embarked on a rigorous treatment plan that included surgeries and chemotherapy. The road was arduous, and there were moments when she felt overwhelmed and disheartened. But she never lost her resilience. Khloe's love for life and her passion for gardening became the driving force behind her determination to conquer the illness that threatened to steal her dreams.

During her chemotherapy sessions, she would visualize her body as a garden, with every powerful medication acting as a gardener, weeding out the cancer cells so that her flowers could bloom once again. This visualization brought her a sense of peace and helped her endure the painful side effects of the treatment.

Khloe's story spread throughout the town, and soon, she became a beacon of hope and inspiration for others fighting similar battles. Strangers sent her letters of encouragement, sharing their own stories of triumph over adversity. She discovered a newfound purpose in connecting with others, offering them solace and hope during their darkest moments.

As the seasons changed, so did Khloe's spirit. The winter of her illness was slowly giving way to the warmth of spring. The pain in her abdomen diminished, and her energy returned little by little. With each passing day, Khloe's flowers bloomed brighter, mirroring her own journey of resilience and renewal.

In the face of adversity, Khloe not only fought ovarian cancer, but she also cultivated a garden of strength, love, and compassion in her heart. Her unwavering determination and indomitable spirit became a testament to the power of hope and the strength that lies within each of us.

And so, as the sun continued to rise and set over the tranquil town, Khloe's story became a living reminder that even amidst life's darkest storms, the human spirit can emerge victorious with love, support, and the will to embrace life's challenges with unwavering courage.

CHAPTER 1

OVERVIEW OF OVARIAN CANCER

UNDERSTANDING OVARIAN CANCER

The reproductive organs in women responsible for creating eggs and hormones—the ovaries—are the site of origin for one particular type of cancer. In women, it is one of the most prevalent types of cancer, and if it is not identified and treated in a timely manner, it may be fatal.

In order to understand ovarian cancer, keep in mind the following:

There are various ovarian cancer subtypes, with epithelial ovarian cancer being the most prevalent. Additionally, there are small cell carcinomas, stromal tumors, and germ cell tumors.

Ovarian cancer risk factors: A few things can make you more likely to get the disease. These include a personal history of breast, colorectal, or uterine cancer, certain medical problems like endometriosis, specific gene mutations (including BRCA1 and BRCA2), growing older, and a family history of ovarian or breast cancer.

SYMPTOMS: Ovarian cancer is frequently called the "silent killer" due to the fact that its signs and symptoms are frequently hazy and can be confused with those of other diseases. Anxiety, exhaustion, changes in bowel habits, frequent urination, stomach bloating or swelling, pelvic pain, feeling full quickly, and unexplained weight loss are common symptoms.

The diagnosis of ovarian cancer usually involves a physical examination, imaging tests (such as an ultrasound, CT scan, or MRI), and blood tests to check for tumor markers like CA-125. A biopsy, a surgical technique where a sample of tissue is removed for analysis, is typically used to provide a certain diagnosis.

Based on the severity of the illness, ovarian cancer is staged. The staging system directs treatment choices and assists in determining how far cancer has spread. From stage I, which is limited to the ovaries, to stage IV, which has spread to other organs, it has four stages.

Surgical removal of the affected tissue, chemotherapy, radiation therapy, and targeted therapy are all possible treatments for ovarian cancer. The stage and kind of cancer, general health, and personal preferences are only a few of the variables that affect the treatment option.

A variety of factors, including the stage of the disease at diagnosis, affect the prognosis for ovarian cancer. Early diagnosis and treatment greatly increase the likelihood of effective therapy and long-term survival.

Ovarian cancer can be difficult to cure and has a higher fatality rate than certain other cancers, however, because symptoms are frequently hazy and diagnosis may come when the disease is too advanced.

Care After Treatment: It's critical to schedule routine follow-up appointments with medical professionals to check for any issues or signs of recurrence after treatment. These visits could involve physical examinations, imaging studies, and blood testing.

RISK ELEMENTS AND PREVENTATIVE MEASURES

Multiple risk factors make ovarian cancer a complicated disease. The risk of ovarian cancer can be increased or decreased by a number of factors, while it is not always possible to prevent it. The following are some of the main ovarian cancer risk factors and possible mitigations:

Hazard Variables

1. Your age: After menopause, especially, your chance of developing ovarian cancer rises with age.

2. A first-degree family (like a mother, sister, or daughter) who has the disease increases the risk.

3. Gene mutations that are passed down from parents: Ovarian cancer risk is greatly increased by mutations in particular genes, such as BRCA1 and BRCA2.

4. Personal history of colorectal or breast cancer: Women who have had colorectal or breast cancer are more likely to acquire ovarian cancer.

5. Hormone replacement therapy (HRT): Using estrogen-only HRT without progesterone for an extended period of time may raise your risk of developing ovarian cancer.

6. Obesity: A person's risk of having ovarian cancer is enhanced if they are overweight or obese.

7. Past pregnancies: Women who have never been pregnant or who became pregnant for the first time after the age of 35 are at higher risk.

8. Endometriosis: Women who have this disorder, in which the uterine lining tissue grows outside the uterus, may be at higher risk.

Measures to Prevent:

1. Oral contraceptives have been demonstrated to lower the incidence of ovarian cancer when used long-term (as in birth control pills). Whether this is a good choice for you to pursue should be discussed with your healthcare professional.

2. Pregnancy and breastfeeding: These two life events lessen a woman's lifetime ovulatory cycle, which lowers her risk of developing ovarian cancer.

3. Tubal ligation or hysterectomy: Surgical procedures like tubal ligation, which involves having your tubes tied, or hysterectomy, which involves removing your uterus, can reduce your risk of developing ovarian cancer, especially if the ovaries are also removed.

4. Genetic counseling and testing: If you have a significant family history of ovarian or breast cancer, especially one linked to BRCA1 or BRCA2 gene mutations, genetic counseling and testing can help you determine your risk and assist you choose the best preventive treatments.

5. Leading a healthy lifestyle: Keeping a healthy weight, eating a balanced diet high in fruits and vegetables, exercising frequently, and giving up smoking may all help lower the risk of developing ovarian cancer.

WARNINGS AND SYMPTOMS

Because the symptoms are sometimes vague and can be mistaken for other common disorders, ovarian cancer can be difficult to identify in its early stages. But it's crucial to remain alert to any possible symptoms or indicators that could point to ovarian cancer. A few of these include

1. Pelvic or abdominal pain: This type of pain, which is frequently described as dull or painful and persistent or frequent, originates in the abdominal or pelvic region.

2. Prolonged bloating or feeling full right away: Even after consuming a tiny amount of food, you may experience prolonged bloating or fullness.

3. Changes in bowel habits: Unexpected variations in bowel movements, such as constipation or diarrhea.

4. Changes in urine habits, such as more frequent urination or difficulties completely emptying the bladder, or increased need to urinate are urinary symptoms.

5. Appetite loss or unexplained weight loss: Sudden loss of appetite or accidental weight loss without a known reason.

6. Fatigue: Ongoing, undiagnosed fatigue that persists despite adequate rest.

7. Constant indigestion, nausea, or discomfort in the lower stomach region.

Back discomfort, often known as lower backache, is a chronic or persistent pain that does not result from an injury or strenuous activity.

9. Menstrual changes: Unusual alterations in menstrual cycles, including heavier or more frequent periods.

It's important to keep in mind that these symptoms can also be brought on by other disorders or illnesses, so just because you have one or more of them does not always suggest you have ovarian cancer.

DIAGNOSTIC TECHNIQUES

The evaluation of a patient's medical history, a physical exam, imaging studies, and laboratory tests are frequently combined in the diagnosis process for ovarian cancer. Following are a few typical methods for ovarian cancer diagnosis:

1. Medical history and physical exam: The physician will inquire about your signs and symptoms, medical background, and any risk factors for ovarian cancer. To look for any anomalies, they will also perform a pelvic examination.

2. Transvaginal ultrasound: This imaging procedure employs sound waves to provide fine-grained pictures of the ovaries. For sharper views of the ovaries and other pelvic tissues, a tiny ultrasound probe is placed into the vagina.

3. Blood test for CA-125: CA-125, a tumor marker, may be increased in ovarian cancer patients. The CA-125 protein in the blood is measured by this blood test. It's crucial to keep in mind, though, that CA-125 levels can also be raised in other diseases, making this test inconclusive in determining whether or not someone has ovarian cancer.

4. Imaging studies: Other imaging tests, such as computed tomography (CT) scans, magnetic resonance imaging (MRI), or positron emission tomography (PET) scans, may be carried out to assess the disease's severity and spot any organ spread.

5. Biopsy: To make a conclusive diagnosis of ovarian cancer, a biopsy is required. From the ovary or any other questionable sites, a small sample of tissue is taken for microscopic analysis. The biopsy can be done surgically, such as during a laparoscopy or laparotomy, or it can be done with the aid of image-guiding methods, such as an ultrasound or CT-guided biopsy.

6. Exploratory surgery: If imaging and other tests indicate ovarian cancer, the doctor may occasionally advise exploratory surgery to visually examine the ovaries, collect tissue samples for a biopsy, and assess the severity of the disease.

STAGING AND PROGNOSIS

It is possible to assess the severity and distribution of ovarian cancer inside the body by staging the disease. It aids medical professionals in deciding on the best course of action and determining a patient's prognosis. The International Federation of Gynecology and Obstetrics (FIGO) staging system is the one that is most frequently used for ovarian cancer. The following phases are included:

Stage I: The ovaries are the only organs affected by the malignancy.

IA: There is just one ovary affected by the malignancy.
The two ovaries are affected by the cancer, IB.

2. Stage II: Other pelvic structures have been affected by the cancer's spread.

The uterus or fallopian tubes are affected by the cancer, according to IIA.
IIB: The bladder or rectum have become affected, as well as other pelvic organs.

3. Stage III: The tumor is still located in the abdomen, but it has progressed to the pelvis.

IIIA: There are tiny cancer cells present in the abdomen and the malignancy has spread to the peritoneum's (the stomach's lining) surface or the ovaries/fallopian tubes.

The peritoneal surfaces bigger than 2 cm in diameter have been affected by the malignancy, according to stage IIIB.

peritoneal surfaces and/or lymph nodes have been affected by the malignancy, according to stage IIIC.

4. Stage IV: The tumor has metastasized to distant organs outside the abdomen.

The liver has been affected by the cancer's spread.

IVB: The cancer has migrated to distant organs like the lungs.

The prognosis of ovarian cancer is influenced by a number of other factors in addition to staging, including:

1. Tumor classification: Under a microscope, the similarity of an ovarian cancer to healthy ovarian tissue determines the tumour's classification. The prognosis is often poorer for high-grade cancers than for low-grade tumors, which also develop more quickly.

2. Tumor histology: Ovarian cancer can be classified into a variety of histological subgroups, such as epithelial, germ cell, and stromal tumors. Every subtype differs from the others in terms of traits and treatment receptivity.

3. Patient's age and general health: The patient's age and general health can influence the prognosis and their capacity to tolerate particular treatments.

4. Treatment response: The prognosis can also be affected by the way the body reacts to the initial course of treatment, including surgery and chemotherapy.

The prognosis can vary greatly depending on these characteristics, and it's crucial to remember that every case is unique. For individualized information and advice about the staging and prognosis of ovarian cancer, it is advised that you speak with a healthcare expert.

TREATMENT OPTIONS

The type and stage of the ovarian cancer, the patient's general health, and their preferences all play a role in the decision of treatment. Listed below are a few typical ovarian cancer treatments:

- **Surgery**: The mainstay of ovarian cancer treatment is typically surgery. The stage and spread of the cancer will determine how much surgery is required. The major objective is to remove all malignant tissue, including the uterus, fallopian tubes, ovaries, and adjacent lymph nodes.

- **Chemotherapy:** This treatment employs medication to destroy cancer cells.

Neoadjuvant chemotherapy shrinks tumors before surgery, whereas adjuvant chemotherapy eliminates any cancer cells that may still be present after surgery. For advanced or reoccurring ovarian cancer, chemotherapy can also be utilized as the main treatment.

- **Targeted Therapy:** Drugs used in targeted therapy selectively target cancer cells while inflicting less damage to healthy cells. They operate by obstructing particular chemicals implicated in the development of cancer. Certain targeted medicines, especially for tumors with particular genetic abnormalities, are approved for use in the treatment of ovarian cancer.

- **Immunotherapy**: Immunotherapy works to amplify the body's immune system's capacity to identify and eliminate cancer cells. When treating specific types of ovarian cancer, it may be used alone or in clinical studies.

- Hormone Therapy: Certain ovarian cancers that are hormone-sensitive are treated with hormone therapy. In this process, hormones that encourage the growth of cancer are blocked or their levels are lowered using drugs.

High-energy X-rays or other particles are used in radiation treatment to eliminate cancer cells. It is not frequently used as the first line of treatment for ovarian cancer, but it may be in some circumstances, such as palliative care to reduce symptoms or targeted treatment of certain locations.

CHAPTER 2

TYPES AND SUBTYPES OVARIAN CANCER

Cancer Of The Ovarian Epithelium

In the epithelial cells, which make up the top layer of cells lining the surface of the ovaries, epithelial ovarian cancer is a form of cancer that develops. Although it can affect women of all ages, menopausal women are predominantly affected by this type of ovarian cancer, which is the most frequent variety.

Epithelial ovarian cancer's precise cause is unknown, although a number of risk factors could make the condition more likely to manifest. Among these danger variables are:

Age: As a woman gets older, her risk of ovarian cancer rises, with most cases affecting those over 50.

Family history: The likelihood of having ovarian cancer is increased in women who have a history of breast, colorectal, or ovarian cancer in their families.

Gene mutations that are inherited: The chance of developing ovarian and breast cancer is considerably increased by mutations in the BRCA1 and BRCA2 genes.

Hormone replacement therapy (HRT): Long-term use of hormone replacement therapy, especially estrogen-only therapy, may tiniest raise the risk of ovarian cancer.

Endometriosis: Women who have the disorder endometriosis, in which the uterine lining tissue protrudes beyond the uterus, are at higher risk of getting ovarian cancer.

Ovarian cancer symptoms can vary depending on how far along it is in the disease. The following symptoms could manifest as the condition worsens:

1. Bloating or swelling inside the stomach

3. Having difficulties eating or experiencing pain or discomfort in the pelvis

4. Modifications to bowel movements, including constipation or more frequent urination

Five. Tired

6. An unforeseen loss or gain in weight

7. Low back ache

8. Uneven menstruation

Diagnosis: If ovarian cancer is suspected, a variety of tests and procedures may be utilized to identify the condition and gauge its severity. One of these is:

During the pelvic exam, the physician looks for any anomalies in the ovaries or the structures around.

Imaging tests like an ultrasound, CT scan, or MRI can help see the ovaries and find any lumps or cancers.

Blood tests: Ovarian cancer may be accompanied by high levels of several blood markers, such as CA-125.

By performing a biopsy, it is possible to determine whether cancer cells are present in the ovaries or adjacent organs.

Surgery and chemotherapy are frequently used as part of the treatment for epithelial ovarian cancer. The particular course of treatment will depend on the cancer's stage, the patient's general health, and other unique considerations.

There are several possible treatments:

- Operative removal of the tumor, ovaries, fallopian tubes, and surrounding lymph nodes is the main course of treatment for ovarian cancer. Debulking surgery is performed in more complex instances with the goal of removing the greatest amount of the tumor.

- **Chemotherapy**: To eliminate any leftover cancer cells after surgery, chemotherapy is frequently given. Chemotherapy for intraperitoneal tumors can be administered intravenously or directly into the abdominal cavity.

- **Targeted therapy:** In some cases of ovarian cancer, medicines that selectively target cancer cells with specific genetic abnormalities may be helpful.

- **Radiation therapy:** Although it is less frequently used in the treatment of ovarian cancer, it may be utilized in rare circumstances.

GERM CELL TUMORS

Obstetrical cancer Ovarian cancers of the germ cell variety—the cells that develop into eggs or ova—are one subtype of the disease. A 15% to 20% proportion of all ovarian malignancies are germ cell tumors.

Both benign and malignant cancers are possible in these lesions. Additional subtype classifications for malignant germ cell tumors include:

The malignant germ cell tumor of the ovary with the highest frequency is called a dysgerminoma. When detected and treated early, it often affects young women and has a favorable prognosis.

In children and young women, endodermal sinus tumors (also known as yolk sac tumors) are more prevalent. Alpha-fetoprotein (AFP), which is frequently produced by it and can be seen in blood tests, is one of its products.

The ovarian germ cell tumor known as an embryonic carcinoma is uncommon and aggressive. It has a quick rate of growth and can invade different body regions.

A positive pregnancy test can be caused by the extremely rare germ cell tumor known as choriocarcinoma, which can also generate hormones associated to pregnancy. It can spread to other organs and is quite aggressive.

Teratoma: This particular type of germ cell tumor, which can either be benign (mature) or malignant (immature), contains a variety of distinct cell types.

In addition to stomach pain or discomfort, bloating, changes in bowel habits, frequent urination, exhaustion, and weight loss, ovarian germ cell tumors can also present with comparable symptoms to other ovarian malignancies.

A biopsy of the tumor is required to confirm the diagnosis of ovarian germ cell tumors. Imaging techniques, such as ultrasound or MRI, blood tests, and tumor markers like AFP and human chorionic gonadotropin, or hCG, are all used in the diagnosis of these tumors.

The kind, stage, and severity of the disease determine the available treatments for ovarian germ cell tumors. Surgical removal of the tumor with the purpose of preserving fertility is frequently the main course of treatment. Chemotherapy may be advised in some situations, especially when a tumor has progressed outside of the ovary.

Depending on the exact subtype, illness stage, and individual circumstances, the prognosis for ovarian germ cell tumors varies. With excellent survival rates in many situations, early discovery and timely treatment can generally result in positive outcomes.

STROMAL TUMORS

Obstetrical cancer A class of uncommon ovarian cancers known as stromal tumors arise from the ovarian stroma, the connective tissue that supports the ovary. Stromal tumors are also referred to as ovarian stromal tumors. Stromal tumors develop from the ovarian cells that make hormones, as opposed to the most prevalent type of ovarian cancer, epithelial ovarian cancer.

Ovarian stromal tumors are primarily of three different types:

1. Granulosa cell tumors: The bulk of ovarian stromal tumors are composed of these lesions, which often affect adults. The granulosa cells, which generate estrogen, give rise to them. Adult and adolescent granulosa cell tumors are two subtypes of granulosa cell tumors, respectively. Due to their propensity to be discovered at an earlier stage, adult granulosa cell tumors typically have a better prognosis than other types of ovarian cancer.

2. Sertoli-Leydig cell tumors: These rare tumors, which mostly affect young women, offer a second option. They are formed from cells that generate androgens, or male hormones. Sertoli-Leydig cell tumors can lead to hormonal abnormalities and symptoms including masculinization or virilization, including the emergence of secondary male sexual traits.

3. Thecoma-fibroma group: This category contains tumors that have features in common with both thecomas and fibromas, which are frequently grouped together. The majority of postmenopausal women experience them; they are mostly benign. Atypical vaginal bleeding is one of the symptoms that thecomas and fibromas, which produce hormones, can induce.

Combining imaging tests (such ultrasound or MRI) with a biopsy to look at the tumor tissue is how ovarian stromal tumors are diagnosed. The tumor's precise nature and stage, as well as the patient's general health, will determine the available treatments. The tumor and surrounding tissues are often removed via surgery, which is the main therapeutic strategy. Chemotherapy or hormonal therapy may be suggested in some circumstances as supplementary treatments.

Ovarian stromal tumors are unique and relatively uncommon, it's vital to remember that.

BORDERLINE OVARIAN TUMORS

Ovarian tumors with low malignant potential (LMP tumors), often referred to as borderline ovarian tumors, are a subtype of ovarian tumor whose behavior falls in between that of benign and malignant tumors. While they share malignant ovarian tumors' aggressive invasion of nearby tissues and dissemination to other areas of the body, benign ovarian tumors are distinguished by aberrant cell development in the ovaries.

An overview of borderline ovarian tumors is provided below.

Ovarian tumors that are borderline are grouped together as a separate subgroup. They differ from both benign and malignant tumors, such as ovarian cancer and cystadenomas. Despite not being invasive, they exhibit several malignancy-related traits.

Behavior: Although it's uncommon, borderline ovarian tumors might return or expand to other areas of the abdomen. They typically stay in the pelvis or the ovary, where they are localized.

During normal pelvic exams or imaging procedures, these tumors are frequently found by accident. The ovary may show them as solid tumors or cystic masses. The tumor may need to be surgically removed for a pathological evaluation or a biopsy may be used to confirm the diagnosis.

Borderline ovarian cancers may not always present with particular symptoms. Some women, however, may feel bloated, have changes in their urine patterns, or endure abdominal pain or discomfort. These symptoms are not unique and can also be present with other ovarian disorders.

Surgical excision of the tumor is the main course of action for borderline ovarian tumors. The size, location, and extent of the tumor, among other things, will determine how extensive the operation will be. Most of the time, fertility-saving surgery is possible, leaving the uterus and unaffected ovary intact if desired. More extensive surgery or chemotherapy may be advised in cases with severe disease or recurrence.

Overall prognosis is good for borderline ovarian tumors. A 5-year survival rate of better than 90% is achieved by the vast majority of women with these malignancies, indicating excellent long-term survival rates. A modest chance of recurrence or development into aggressive cancer needs close follow-up, nonetheless.

Care after treatment: To identify any signs of recurrence or advancement, it's crucial to have regular follow-up appointments and monitoring. This may involve physical examinations, blood tests (such as CA-125), and imaging studies.

RARE OVARIAN CANCERS

A group of cancerous tumors that develop in the ovaries on an occasional basis are referred to as rare ovarian malignancies. Although epithelial ovarian carcinomas account for the bulk of ovarian malignancies, there are a number of uncommon histological forms of ovarian cancer that are also rare. Comparing these uncommon forms to the more prevalent epithelial ovarian tumors, it is frequently clear that they have different traits, therapeutic strategies, and prognoses.

Instances of uncommon ovarian malignancies include the following:

Germ cell tumors: These cancers arise from the cells that make eggs. Only 5% of ovarian malignancies are caused by them. There are two types of germ cell tumors: benign and malignant. Malignant germ cell tumors can take various forms, such as dysgerminoma, yolk sac tumor, embryonal carcinoma, choriocarcinoma, and teratoma.

Sex cord-stramal tumors: These tumors develop from the cells that assemble the ovaries and make female hormones. About 1% of ovarian malignancies are caused by them. Tumors with Sertoli-Leydig cells and granulosa cells are two examples.

Ovarian small cell carcinoma: Ovarian small cell carcinoma is a very uncommon and aggressive form of the disease that usually affects young females. It has a high potential for metastasis and is distinguished by tiny, rounded cells.

Mucinous Carcinoma: Mucinous carcinoma is a form of ovarian epithelial cancer, but it is uncommon in comparison to serous carcinomas, which are much more typical. Mucus production is the defining characteristic of mucinous carcinomas, which can also feature gastrointestinal and endocervical-like subtypes.

Clear Cell Carcinoma: A tiny proportion of ovarian malignancies are caused by this additional subtype of epithelial ovarian cancer. In comparison to other ovarian cancer types, it frequently resists chemotherapy and has a worse prognosis.

A uncommon, aggressive tumor that combines carcinomatous (epithelial) and sarcomatous (mesenchymal) components is referred to as a carcinosarcoma (Malignant Mixed Müllerian Tumor). The prognosis is generally bad and it is frequently detected at an advanced stage.

It is crucial to remember that each of these uncommon ovarian cancers has distinct characteristics, such as various development patterns, genetic changes, and responses to therapy. Due to their rarity, unique treatment methods and knowledge may be necessary, and patients are frequently managed in specialized centers with experience handling rare gynecologic malignancies.

CHAPTER 3

PATHOGENESIS AND GENETICS OVARIAN CANCER

Genetic Mutations and Susceptibility

Complex genetic and environmental factors interact to affect the development of ovarian cancer. Although it's vital to keep in mind that not all occurrences of ovarian cancer are brought on by genetic abnormalities, they can enhance one's vulnerability to the disease. In actuality, the majority of occurrences of ovarian cancer are sporadic and lack a definite genetic inheritance.

Having said that, various genetic changes have been recognized as ovarian cancer risk factors. BRCA1 and BRCA2 mutations are the most popular and in-depth researched genetic abnormalities linked to ovarian cancer. Only a small proportion of ovarian cancer cases—roughly 10-15%—are thought to be caused by these mutations, which are inherited in an autosomal dominant pattern.

Comparatively to the general population, women who inherit mutant BRCA1 or BRCA2 genes are far more likely to develop ovarian cancer. But it's crucial to remember that these mutations also raise the risk of other diseases, like breast cancer. Furthermore, not everyone with BRCA1 or BRCA2 mutations will have ovarian cancer, suggesting that additional variables may affect disease development.

Though these mutations are very uncommon, ovarian cancer risk has been linked to other gene mutations besides BRCA1 and BRCA2, despite the fact that they are less common. TP53, PTEN, and mismatch repair genes, which are linked to Lynch syndrome and Li-Fraumeni syndrome, respectively, are a few examples of genes having mutations.

It's crucial to keep in mind that the existence of these mutations just raises the vulnerability to the disease rather than ensuring that it will manifest. The emergence of ovarian cancer is also influenced by a wide range of additional factors, including hormonal factors, environmental exposures, lifestyle decisions, and chance.

It is advised to speak with a healthcare provider or genetic counselor if you have concerns about your individual risk of developing ovarian cancer or any other health-related issues. These individuals may offer individualized information and advice based on your unique circumstances.

MOLECULAR PATHWAYS

The genesis and progression of ovarian cancer is a complicated illness that is influenced by numerous molecular pathways. The molecular mechanisms linked to ovarian cancer will be thoroughly outlined here:

1. DNA Damage Response and Repair Pathway: Errors in DNA repair pathways can result in an accumulation of genetic mutations and genomic instability, which aids in the growth of ovarian cancer. DNA repair is facilitated by a number of pathways, including the homologous recombination (HR) route, nucleotide excision repair (NER), base excision repair (BER), and mismatch repair (MMR).

2. Cell Cycle Regulation Pathway: Dysregulation of the cell cycle control systems can cause unchecked cell growth and division, which is a defining feature of cancer. Important cell cycle regulators include cyclins, cyclin-dependent kinases (CDKs), and tumor suppressor proteins including p53 and retinoblastoma (RB). Ovarian cancer development may be aided by abnormalities in these pathways.

3. The PI3K/AKT/mTOR Signaling Pathway: This pathway controls metabolism, cell growth, proliferation, and survival. In ovarian cancer, dysregulation of the phosphatidylinositol 3-kinase (PI3K)/AKT/mammalian target of rapamycin (mTOR) pathway is frequently seen and has been linked to tumor growth, angiogenesis, and treatment resistance.

4. Wnt/-catenin Signaling Pathway: In ovarian cancer, aberrant activation of the Wnt/-catenin pathway can encourage tumor development and progression. The stabilization and nuclear translocation of -catenin, which results in the transcriptional activation of Wnt target genes, can be caused by mutations in important elements of this pathway, such as -catenin or adenomatous polyposis coli (APC).

5. Notch Signaling Pathway: Notch signaling is essential for cell proliferation, survival, and destiny determination. Ovarian cancer development and progression have been linked to dysregulation of the Notch system. Angiogenesis can be boosted, apoptosis is inhibited, and cell proliferation is promoted by abnormal Notch signaling activity.

6. The TGF- Signaling Pathway Transforming growth factor-beta (TGF-) signaling controls a number of biological functions, such as cell division, proliferation, apoptosis, and immune response. The growth, metastasis, and refractoriness of ovarian cancer have all been linked to altered TGF- signaling, which can either lose responsiveness or gain function.

7.The Pathway of Epithelial-Mesenchymal Transition (EMT): Epithelial cells acquire a mesenchymal character through the dynamic process of EMT. Tumor invasion, metastasis, and treatment resistance are all significantly influenced by EMT. Snail, Slug, and Twist are important transcription factors involved in EMT that can be induced by a number of signaling pathways, including TGF- and Wnt/-catenin.

8. Angiogenesis Pathway: The development of new blood vessels, or angiogenesis, is crucial for the growth and spread of tumors. In the angiogenesis pathway, vascular endothelial growth factor (VEGF) and its receptors (VEGFRs) are important actors. Ovarian cancer frequently exhibits overexpression of VEGF and enhanced angiogenesis.

These are some of the molecular pathways connected to ovarian cancer, but it's crucial to remember that ovarian cancer formation and progression are multifactorial and include an intricate interaction of many molecular processes.

EFFECTS OF HORMONES AND THE ENVIRONMENT

A number of hormonal and environmental factors can affect the development of the complex disease ovarian cancer. Detailed hormonal and environmental factors linked to ovarian cancer include the following:

Hormonal Influences

- Age of Menarche and Menopause: Early menarche and late menopause increase lifetime exposure to ovarian hormones like estrogen, which may help to increase the risk of ovarian cancer.

- **Hormone Replacement Therapy (HRT):** Long-term usage of estrogen-only HRT has been linked to an increased risk of ovarian cancer, particularly when progesterone is not used.

- Oral Contraceptives: It has been discovered that using birth control tablets can lower your risk of developing ovarian cancer. The preventive impact grows stronger the longer it is used, and the risk decrease lasts for several years after it is stopped.

- Pregnancy and Parity: Studies have linked numerous births and full-term pregnancies to a lower risk of ovarian cancer. The temporary inhibition of ovulation and variations in hormone levels during pregnancy may be responsible for the protective effect.

- Infertility and Fertility Treatments: Ovarian cancer may be increased by infertility in and of itself. Certain fertility procedures, such ovulation-inducing medications (like clomiphene citrate) or in vitro fertilization (IVF), may marginally raise the risk, according to certain research. To establish a clear correlation, more investigation is necessary.

Environmental Influences

1. Family History and Genetic Factors: Breast and ovarian cancer risk are considerably increased by inherited gene mutations, such as those in the BRCA1 and BRCA2 genes. Additional genetic syndromes that increase risk include Lynch syndrome and hereditary nonpolyposis colorectal cancer (HNPCC).

2. Personal History of Cancer: An increased risk of ovarian cancer results from a prior diagnosis of breast, colorectal, or endometrial cancer.

3. Environmental Toxins: Exposure to several environmental toxins and chemicals, like asbestos, talc, pesticides, and industrial chemicals like polychlorinated biphenyls (PCBs), may raise the risk of ovarian cancer. The precise mechanisms, however, are still being researched.

4. Obesity: Being overweight or obese has been associated to a higher risk of ovarian cancer, which may be brought on by higher amounts of the estrogen produced by fat cells, ongoing inflammation, and insulin resistance.

5. Lifestyle Factors: Smoking, binge drinking, eating poorly balanced diets devoid of fruits and vegetables, and other lifestyle choices may all raise the risk of developing ovarian cancer.

It's crucial to remember that while these variables may affect the likelihood of getting ovarian cancer, they do not ensure the disease will manifest itself. These factors interact in a complex way, and each case will be different. Accurate risk assessment and early detection depend on routine screenings, genetic testing (where appropriate), and competent medical advice.

OVARIAN CANCER AND INFLAMMATION

Inflammation is the body's intricate biochemical response to noxious stimuli like infections, wounds, and autoimmune diseases. Although inflammation is an essential component of the body's defensive system, chronic or persistent inflammation can speed up the onset and spread of many illnesses, including cancer. Ovarian cancer, which affects the ovaries, a component of the female reproductive system, is a particularly severe type of cancer. The connection between inflammation and ovarian cancer is examined in this article, along with any relevant processes, risk factors, diagnostic indicators, and treatment implications.

INFLAMMATION AND THE DEVELOPMENT OF OVARIAN CANCER

There is growing evidence that chronic inflammation may be a major factor in the development and spread of ovarian cancer. The hallmarks of the development of cancer, including DNA damage, genomic instability, cell proliferation, angiogenesis (the formation of new blood vessels), and immune suppression, can all be facilitated by inflammatory processes. Prostaglandins, cytokines, and chemokines are examples of inflammatory mediators that can produce an inflammatory microenvironment that supports the growth and survival of cancer cells.

Ovarian cancer and inflammatory processes: There are a number of theories put forth to explain the link between inflammation and ovarian cancer. These consist of:

Pro-inflammatory pathways can be activated, which can result in an increase in cell proliferation, survival, and angiogenesis. Examples of these signaling pathways include NF-B (nuclear factor-kappa B), STAT3 (signal transducer and activator of transcription 3), and COX-2 (cyclooxygenase-2).

b. Genomic instability and DNA damage: Inflammatory processes produce reactive oxygen and nitrogen species that can damage DNA and result in genetic mutations, raising the risk of the development of ovarian cancer.

c. **Modulation of the immune system:** Prolonged inflammation can impair the immune system's capacity to identify and destroy cancer cells, allowing them to grow unchecked.

Risk Factors and Inflammatory Diseases: Some risk factors and inflammatory diseases have been linked to an increased risk of ovarian cancer development. These consist of:

A chronic inflammatory state is exacerbated by obesity, which causes adipose tissue to produce pro-inflammatory cytokines.

b. Endometriosis: This condition, which involves endometrial tissue existing outside the uterus, is linked to increased inflammation and an increased risk of ovarian cancer.

c. Pelvic inflammatory disease (PID): Chronic pelvic inflammation brought on by infections, such as STDs, has been associated with a higher risk of ovarian cancer.

d. Aging: Chronic low-grade inflammation in older women has been linked to an increased risk of ovarian cancer.

Inflammatory markers have demonstrated potential as diagnostic and prognostic indicators for ovarian cancer. Advanced stages of ovarian cancer have been linked to higher levels of C-reactive protein (CRP), interleukin-6 (IL-6), and tumor necrosis factor-alpha (TNF-alpha), as well as worse outcomes. These markers' measurement could help with prognosis prediction, early detection, and treatment response monitoring.

Targeting pathways and mediators connected to inflammation may be a new therapeutic strategy for treating ovarian cancer. In preclinical and clinical studies, a number of anti-inflammatory drugs, such as nonsteroidal anti-inflammatory drugs (NSAIDs), COX-2 inhibitors, and immunomodulatory drugs, have demonstrated promise. Immunotherapies, which improve the immune system's capacity to identify and destroy cancer cells, are also being investigated as potential therapeutic approaches.

The onset and spread of ovarian cancer are significantly influenced by chronic inflammation. Knowing the mechanisms underlying the relationship between inflammation and ovarian cancer can help identify potential therapeutic targets and diagnostic indicators.

CHAPTER 4

DETECTION AND EARLY SCREENING

Modern Screening Techniques

Here are some of the most recent ovarian cancer screening procedures:

- **Transvaginal ultrasound (TVUS):** With this technique, an ultrasound probe is inserted into the vagina to produce images of the ovaries. It can aid in locating any ovarian abnormalities or masses that might need further examination.

- **CA-125 Blood Test:** Some ovarian cancer patients may have elevated levels of the protein CA-125 in their blood. This blood test measures the CA-125 levels and serves as a potential ovarian cancer marker. However, the specificity of CA-125 is limited because it can also be elevated in non-cancerous conditions.

- Risk assessment and family history: Determining the need for additional screening or genetic testing can be aided by assessing a woman's risk factors for ovarian cancer, such as her family's history of the condition or particular genetic mutations (such as BRCA1 and BRCA2).

- Pelvic Exam: In a pelvic exam, a medical professional visually inspects a woman's reproductive organs, including her ovaries, to look for any abnormalities or masses. However, this approach by itself is not regarded as a reliable screening tool for ovarian cancer in its early stages.

- Combination Approaches: To increase the efficacy of ovarian cancer detection, some studies are investigating the use of a combination of screening techniques. For instance, combining TVUS with the blood test for CA-125 or other biomarkers may improve the screening procedure.

It's significant to remember that there is currently no widely accepted screening procedure for ovarian cancer in the general population. This is primarily due to the sensitivity, specificity, and cost-effectiveness limitations of the screening techniques currently in use. In addition, ovarian cancer is frequently discovered in advanced stages, when it has already spread outside the ovaries.

EARLY DETECTION CHALLENGES

1. Generalized symptoms: Ovarian cancer frequently exhibits generalized symptoms like bloating, abdominal pain, fatigue, and frequent urination. It is challenging to detect ovarian cancer at an early stage because these symptoms are frequently linked to other illnesses.

2. Absence of a widely accepted and trustworthy screening test: Unlike breast cancer, which is detectable through mammograms, ovarian cancer does not have such a test. This makes it more challenging to identify the disease early.

3. Silent progression: Ovarian cancer is renowned for its silent progression, which means that it can advance without manifesting any symptoms. It's possible that the cancer has progressed to an advanced stage by the time symptoms start to show.

4. Low disease prevalence: Ovarian cancer is uncommon compared to other cancers, making it difficult to create effective screening programs. It is more challenging to defend widespread screening initiatives given the low prevalence.

5. The absence of specific biomarkers: Biomarkers are substances that can reveal the existence of a disease. There are currently no specific early-stage ovarian cancer biomarkers that are sensitive and specific enough for routine clinical use.

6. Physical constraints: It is challenging to access the ovaries for an examination because they are buried deep within the pelvis. Because of this, tumors are harder to find during routine physical exams.

7. Underdiagnosis and misdiagnosis: Due to the symptoms that ovarian cancer shares with other benign conditions, it is very easy to make a mistaken diagnosis or to overlook it. Underdiagnosis may be influenced by the absence of specific symptoms and valid screening exams.

8. Lack of knowledge: It's possible that both women and medical professionals are under informed about ovarian cancer's early warning signs and symptoms. Delays in diagnosis and lost chances for early detection can be the result of this.

9. Genetic factors: Some cases of ovarian cancer are linked to genetic mutations, such as those in the BRCA1 and BRCA2 genes. It is difficult to determine which women are at a higher risk because not all ovarian cancer patients have these mutations.

10. The prognosis for ovarian cancer significantly improves when it is found at an early stage. There are few treatment options for advanced stages. Unfortunately, because early detection is difficult, a lot of cases are only discovered when they are far along, leaving patients with few options for treatment and less favorable outcomes.

In order to meet these challenges, more work needs to be done on sensitive and precise biomarkers, on the genetics of ovarian cancer, on raising awareness among women and healthcare professionals, and on creating screening programs that are effective and specifically designed for ovarian cancer.

CHAPTER 5

STAGING AND DIAGNOSIS

Techniques for Imaging

In order to accurately diagnose, stage, and plan treatment for ovarian cancer, a variety of imaging techniques are needed. Several imaging procedures for ovarian cancer include the following:

An initial imaging technique frequently used to assess ovarian abnormalities is transvaginal ultrasound (TVUS). To obtain precise images of the ovaries, uterus, and surrounding structures, a tiny ultrasound probe must be inserted into the vagina. TVUS can assist in identifying ovarian masses, classifying their nature (solid or cystic), and determining the tumor's size, location, and vascularity.

Detailed cross-sectional images of the abdomen and pelvis are produced by CT scans, which use a series of X-ray images as their starting point. The spread of the disease, the involvement of the lymph nodes, and the presence of distant metastases can all be determined by CT scans. To make blood vessels and tumors more visible, intravenous contrast may be used.

A strong magnetic field and radio waves are used in magnetic resonance imaging (MRI) to produce precise images of the pelvis and abdomen. It can aid in identifying benign from malignant ovarian masses and offer excellent soft tissue contrast. When analyzing tumor characteristics, the involvement of nearby organs, and lymph node involvement, MRI is especially helpful.

Positron Emission Tomography (PET) Scan: In PET scans, a small quantity of radioactive material is injected into the body. This radioactive material is absorbed by metabolically active cells, such as cancer cells. PET scans can be used to monitor the effectiveness of treatment, look for distant metastases, and look for ovarian cancer recurrence.

Fluorodeoxyglucose (FDG) PET/CT: This type of imaging combines PET and CT. It provides anatomical as well as functional information, assisting in pinpointing the precise location of cancer cells within the body and locating regions of elevated glucose metabolism (indicative of cancer cells).

Ultrasound-Guided Biopsy: Ultrasound-guided biopsies may be used to make a diagnosis when imaging alone is insufficient. During this procedure, a needle is inserted into a tumor or other suspicious area with the help of real-time ultrasound images in order to collect a tissue sample for further examination.

The minimally invasive surgical procedure known as laparoscopy, which allows for direct visualization of the ovaries and surrounding structures, is not technically an imaging technique. It can be applied to the staging of ovarian cancer and the collection of tissue samples for analysis.

It's crucial to remember that the selection of imaging method(s) depends on a number of variables, including the patient's clinical state, the stage of the cancer, and the knowledge and resources offered by the healthcare facility. For each unique case of ovarian cancer, the best imaging methods should be chosen and interpreted by a multidisciplinary team of medical experts, including radiologists, oncologists, and surgeons.

Histopathological evaluation and biopsies

Details about the patient:
Identifier: [Patient Name]
Patient's age at [date]

Identifier: [Patient Gender]
[Patient MRN] is the medical record number.
Date of Biopsy: [Biopsy Date]
Report's release date is [Date of Report].

Clinical History: Based on [clinical findings/examinations], it was suspected that the patient, who presented with [symptoms], had ovarian cancer. The diagnosis was verified through an ovarian tissue biopsy.

Information on the Sample:
Ovarian tissue is the specimen type.
[Left/Right] is the specimen source. The received specimen is an ovary, and it includes [specimen description].

The specimen has [dimensions] according to the macroscopic examination. The ovarian tissue is visible externally and exhibits [characteristics, such as enlargement and irregularity]. Additional macroscopic findings are visible on the cut surface, such as solid areas, necrosis, and hemorrhage.

Microscopic Analysis: The sections that had been stained with H&E underwent microscopic analysis. The sections display [microscopic results].

1. Tumor Type and Grade: The tissue of the ovaries exhibits characteristics consistent with [type of ovarian tumor]. The tumor is classified as [grade, if applicable, e.g., low-grade, high-grade] based on [grading system, if applicable, e.g., FIGO grading system].

2. Tumor Extent and Invasion: The tumor exhibits [involvement of the ovarian tissue, such as focal, multifocal, or diffuse tumor involvement]. There is evidence of invasion within the [structures involved, such as the peritoneum, nearby fallopian tubes, and ovarian stroma].

3. Histological Subtypes: The tumor's histological analysis reveals the existence of [histological subtypes, if applicable, such as

serous, mucinous, endometrioid, and clear cell].

4. Tumor Differentiation: Areas of the tumor exhibit [degree of differentiation, e.g., well-differentiated, moderately differentiated, poorly differentiated].

5. Stromal Reaction: The stroma in the vicinity of the tumor exhibits [stromal reaction features, such as desmoplastic reaction, inflammatory infiltrate].

6. Lymphovascular Invasion: Lymphovascular invasion is found inside the tumor, which raises the possibility of metastatic spread.

Immunohistochemistry: An immunohistochemical analysis was carried out to examine particular markers and further characterize the tumor. Here are the findings:

1 [Marker 1]

Amount: [Positive/Negative]
Weak, moderate, or strong is the intensity.
Availability: [Localized/Diffuse]

2 [Marker 2]:

Amount: [Positive/Negative]
Weak, moderate, or strong is the intensity.
Availability: [Localized/Diffuse]
[Additional markers, if any, should be included]

Ovarian tissue underwent a biopsy and histopathological analysis, and the results showed evidence of ovarian cancer. The ovarian tumor is categorized as having [histological subtypes, if applicable] components. The grade of the tumor is [grade, if applicable]. Within the [involved structures], invasion is evident. The stroma displays [stromal reaction characteristics]. The possibility of metastatic spread is suggested by the discovery of lymphovascular invasion.

Additional molecular investigations, such as genetic analysis and additional ancillary tests, may offer more prognostic and therapeutic data.

Please be aware that this report, which is based on the histopathological analysis of the biopsy specimen, should be interpreted in conjunction with any relevant clinical and radiological findings. To make the best management and treatment choices, clinical correlation is advised.

By: [Pathologist's Name]
Observed on: [Date of Signature]

Disclaimer: This report is a simulated illustration and shouldn't be used in place of a genuine medical report.

Astatic Ascites and Tumor Markers

Ascites and tumor markers for ovarian cancer that are frequently used include:

Analyzing ascites

A microscopic examination of ascitic fluid is known as ascitic fluid cytology, and it is used to detect cancer cells.
A measurement of the protein content of ascitic fluid.
cancer markers

- CA-125 (Cancer Antigen 125): This tumor marker is the most popular one for ovarian cancer. CA-125 can be elevated in other conditions like endometriosis or pelvic inflammatory disease, though elevated levels can also be a sign of ovarian cancer.

In addition to CA-125, HE4 (Human Epididymis Protein 4) is a tumor marker. Detecting ovarian cancer in its earliest stages and keeping track of treatment effectiveness may benefit from it.

- CA 19-9 (Carbohydrate Antigen 19-9): While elevated levels of CA 19-9 have been linked to ovarian cancer, the marker is less specific than CA-125.

- CEA (Carcinoembryonic Antigen): While it is not frequently used as a specific marker for ovarian cancer, CEA levels may be elevated in some cases.

- AFP (Alpha-Fetoprotein): AFP is frequently linked to specific cancers, such as liver tumors and germ cell tumors. The marker does not specifically indicate ovarian cancer.

- Inhibin: Certain ovarian tumor types, like granulosa cell tumors, can exhibit elevated levels of inhibin.

Please remember that ovarian cancer cannot be definitively diagnosed just because these markers are present. Often, a complete diagnosis necessitates additional diagnostic procedures like biopsies and imaging studies (ultrasound, CT scan, MRI).

The FIGO Staging System

To stage ovarian cancer, doctors frequently use the FIGO (International Federation of Gynecology and Obstetrics) staging system. The size of the tumor, the degree of pelvic and abdominal spread, lymph node involvement, and distant metastasis are just a few of the variables that are considered. Here is the ovarian cancer staging system recommended by FIGO:

The ovaries are the only sites of the cancer in stage I.

- IA: The cancer only affects one ovary, and the tumor is only present on the ovary's surface.

Both ovaries are affected by cancer, but the tumor is still contained to the ovarian surfaces.

- IC: The tumor is either stage IA or stage IB, but there are malignant cells on the outer surface of one or both ovaries, or the tumor capsule has ruptured, or the ovary's surface is involved, or there are tumor cells in ascites or peritoneal washings.

Stage II: Additional pelvic structures are affected by the cancer's spread.

The uterus or fallopian tubes are affected by the cancer, according to IIA.

The bladder, rectum, or colon are just a few examples of other pelvic organs where the cancer has metastasized.

Stage III: The abdomen is still affected, but the cancer has spread beyond the pelvis.

- IIIA: There are tiny cancerous deposits in the abdomen beyond the pelvis that are less than 2 cm in size, or the tumor has metastasized to the surface of the liver or spleen.

-;IIIB: The liver, spleen, or abdominal cavity contain tumor implants larger than 2 cm.

The lymph nodes in the abdomen have been affected by cancer, stage IIIC.

Stage IV: The liver or other distant organs have been affected by the cancer's metastases.

IVA: The lung cancer has become more advanced.

- IVB: The cancer has reached additional distant organs, like the bones or the brain.

It's significant to note that this staging system offers a uniform way to group ovarian cancer according to the severity of the condition. In deciding on a course of treatment and estimating prognosis, the stage of ovarian cancer is extremely important.

CHAPTER 6

TREATMENT STRATEGIES

Surgery for Ovarian Cancer

When treating ovarian cancer, surgery is frequently used. A number of variables, including the cancer's stage, the size and location of the tumor, and the patient's general health, will determine the precise surgical procedure. Surgical procedures frequently used to treat ovarian cancer include the following:

One or both ovaries may be removed during an ovarian tumor removal procedure, also known as an oophorectomy. A unilateral oophorectomy, which involves removing just one ovary, is referred to as such, whereas a bilateral oophorectomy involves removing both ovaries. The removal of the lymph nodes close by and the fallopian tubes is a possibility in some circumstances.

Surgery to remove the uterus is called hysterectomy. The extent of the cancer will determine whether the surgeon performs a partial hysterectomy, which involves only the uterus, or a total hysterectomy, which involves both the uterus and cervix. In addition to oophorectomy, hysterectomy is also an option.

Lymph Node Dissection: During surgery, it may be necessary to remove lymph nodes from the pelvis and abdomen to check for the presence of cancer that has spread past the ovaries. Planning for additional treatment is aided by this procedure for staging the cancer.

To remove as much of the tumor as possible, debulking surgery (also known as cytoreduction) is carried out on patients with advanced-stage ovarian cancer. In order to do this, it may be necessary to remove not only the ovaries but also other affected organs or tissues, including the fallopian tubes, the uterus, the omentum (fatty tissue covering the intestines), and some of the colon or bladder.

Laparoscopic Surgery: Minimally invasive laparoscopic surgery for ovarian cancer may be an option in some circumstances. To remove the tumor or carry out other necessary procedures, this technique entails making small incisions and using a camera and specialized surgical tools. Faster recovery, less noticeable scarring, and decreased postoperative pain are all benefits of laparoscopic surgery.

The precise surgical strategy and scope will depend on the case of each patient and the surgeon's evaluation, it is important to note. Treatment for ovarian cancer frequently involves a variety of interdisciplinary approaches, including surgery, chemotherapy, radiation therapy, and targeted therapies. Based on the cancer's stage, characteristics, the patient's general health, and personal preferences, the oncology team decides on a specific treatment strategy.

Chemotherapy Options

ovarian cancer treatment options using chemotherapy. The stage and type of the patient's ovarian cancer, the patient's general health, and the patient's personal preferences as well as those of their medical team may all influence the choice of chemotherapy regimen. For individualized guidance and treatment choices, it's crucial to speak with a licensed oncologist. Given that, the following are a few frequently employed ovarian cancer chemotherapy options:

Chemotherapy with a platinum base: The cornerstone of chemotherapy for ovarian cancer is frequently composed of platinum-based medications like cisplatin and carboplatin. By damaging cancer cells' DNA, these medications prevent the division and growth of cancer cells.

Chemotherapy with a taxane base: Paclitaxel and docetaxel are two examples of taxane drugs that are frequently combined with chemotherapy that uses platinum as the base. In order to disrupt the internal structure and functions of cancer cells, they interfere with the microtubules within those cells.

chemotherapy in combination: Combining chemotherapy with taxane- and platinum-based drugs is the most widely used strategy for treating ovarian cancer. When compared to single-drug therapy, this combination—often referred to as the "platinum-taxane doublet"—has shown improved efficacy.

Chemotherapy may occasionally be administered intraperitoneally (through a catheter) into the peritoneal cavity, which is the space surrounding the abdominal organs. The intraperitoneal chemotherapy method can assist in getting higher drug concentrations to the tumor site.

Alternatively, intravenous chemotherapy may be used in place of it.

The development of targeted therapies for ovarian cancer has recently taken place. Specific molecules or pathways involved in the development and spread of cancer are the focus of these medications. To stop new blood vessels from growing and supplying the tumor with nutrients, for instance, one could use medications like bevacizumab.

It's crucial to keep in mind that the particular chemotherapy plan and length of the course can vary greatly depending on a number of factors. The best course of treatment for you will be decided by your doctor after taking into account a number of variables.

RADIATION THERAPY

When treating ovarian cancer, radiation therapy, also referred to as radiotherapy, may be used. The primary method of treatment for ovarian cancer is not frequently radiation therapy, it is crucial to remember this. Typically, this type of cancer is treated primarily with surgery and chemotherapy.

The following circumstances may call for radiation therapy:

1. Adjuvant radiation therapy: After the tumor has been surgically removed, radiation therapy may be used to kill any cancer cells that may still be present in the pelvic region. Adjuvant radiation therapy is what this is referred to as, and it is employed to lower the risk of cancer recurrence.

2. Palliative radiation therapy: Palliative radiation therapy can be used to treat ovarian cancer that has spread to the bones or the brain in order to lessen symptoms and enhance quality of life. Focused on reducing pain or other cancer-related symptoms, this type of radiation therapy is known as palliative radiation therapy.

Determine the best course of treatment for a specific patient by speaking with an oncologist or radiation oncologist who specializes in the treatment of ovarian cancer. Several variables, including the cancer's stage, the tumor's location, and the patient's general health, will determine whether radiation therapy is necessary.

In order to damage the cancerous cells' DNA and prevent them from proliferating and dividing, radiation therapy involves exposing the cancerous cells to high-energy X-rays or other types of radiation. In order to give healthy cells time to recover between treatments, the treatment is typically given over a period of several weeks during multiple sessions.

Radiation therapy might come with side effects, just like any other cancer treatment. Fatigue, skin changes, nausea, diarrhea, and irritation of the bladder or bowel are a few of these side effects, which vary depending on the area being treated. The radiation oncology staff will keep a close eye on the patient throughout the course of treatment and offer supportive care to treat any side effects.

It is important to discuss treatment options and potential side effects with the medical team managing the patient's care because specifics of the course of treatment will vary depending on the circumstances of each individual case.

TARGETED THERAPIES

The stage and subtype of ovarian cancer will determine the available treatments because it is a complex disease. By specifically focusing on molecules and pathways involved in cancer growth and progression, targeted therapies have emerged as a promising strategy for treating ovarian cancer. Examples of targeted therapies for the treatment of ovarian cancer include the following:

Inhibitors of poly (ADP-ribose) polymerase (PARP), such as olaparib, niraparib, and rucaparib, have demonstrated notable effectiveness in the treatment of ovarian cancer, particularly in patients with BRCA1 or BRCA2 gene mutations. The DNA damage builds up and the cancer cells die as a result of PARP inhibitors' interference with DNA repair mechanisms.

VEGF inhibitors: Vascular endothelial growth factor (VEGF) is a protein that encourages the development of new blood vessels, a process known as angiogenesis. By preventing the growth of new blood vessels in tumors, VEGF inhibition helps to lessen the blood supply to the tumors and slow their growth. In the treatment of advanced ovarian cancer, VEGF inhibitors like bevacizumab have been combined with chemotherapy.

Anti-HER2 treatments: Some ovarian cancers may overexpress human epidermal growth factor receptor 2 (HER2), a protein that encourages cell division and growth. In order to ascertain the efficacy of HER2-targeted therapies in HER2-positive ovarian cancer, clinical trials have been conducted with drugs like trastuzumab.

Anti-angiogenic treatments: Other anti-angiogenic drugs that target various angiogenesis-related signaling pathways are being investigated as alternatives to VEGF inhibitors as ovarian cancer treatments. Inhibitors of multiple angiogenic pathways like cediranib and trebananib are among these.

Immunotherapies: Immune checkpoint inhibitors, such as pembrolizumab and nivolumab, have shown promising results in the treatment of specific types of ovarian cancer. By releasing the immune system's restraints, these medications help the body's defenses more effectively identify and combat cancer cells.

It's important to keep in mind that the availability of targeted therapies may differ depending on the nation and particular healthcare setting. Usually, medical professionals decide whether to use these therapies after carefully examining the patient's unique characteristics, such as tumor biomarkers and genetic mutations, to customize the course of treatment.

IMMUNOTHERAPY

Ovarian cancer is just one of the many types of cancer for which immunotherapy has emerged as a promising treatment option. Often diagnosed at an advanced stage, ovarian cancer is renowned for being challenging to detect and treat. Opioid therapy has shown promise in potentially improving outcomes for some patients, but traditional therapies like surgery, chemotherapy, and radiation therapy have been the mainstay of ovarian cancer treatment for years.

Ovarian cancer immunotherapy is being studied using a variety of approaches, including:

Immune checkpoint inhibitors are a class of medications that block proteins on immune cells or cancer cells that stop the immune system from attacking cancer cells. For some subsets of ovarian cancer patients, particularly those with tumors that have high levels of particular immune cells, checkpoint inhibitors like pembrolizumab and nivolumab have demonstrated promising outcomes in clinical trials.

2. Chimeric Antigen Receptor T-Cell Therapy: In CAR-T therapy, cancer cells are recognized and attacked by a patient's own immune cells (T-cells) that have been modified in a lab to recognize and attack them. While CAR-T therapy has demonstrated remarkable efficacy in treating some blood cancers, its use in solid tumors like ovarian cancer is still being explored

and is still regarded as an active research area.

3. Tumor-infiltrating lymphocytes therapy (TIL therapy): TIL therapy involves removing immune cells from a patient's tumor, isolating and growing them in a lab, and then re-infusing them into the patient. The effectiveness and safety of TIL therapy for ovarian cancer are being examined in clinical trials.

4. Vaccines: Cancer vaccines work to activate the immune system so that it can identify and combat cancer cells. While early clinical trials of some ovarian cancer vaccines, such as the peptide vaccine known as OVA1, showed promise, more studies are required to determine the effectiveness of these vaccines.

Though some ovarian cancer patients have experienced significant benefits from immunotherapy, it's important to remember that not everyone will benefit from it. A positive response to immunotherapy can be predicted by patient characteristics and biomarkers, allowing for more individualized treatment strategies.

When considering immunotherapy for ovarian cancer, as with any medical procedure, it is essential to speak with a medical expert who can give you the most recent information on the various treatment options, clinical trials, and potential advantages and disadvantages of the procedure.

HORMONAL THERAPIES

Because ovarian cancer typically responds better to surgical intervention and chemotherapy, hormonal therapies are not typically the first-line treatment for the condition. Hormonal therapies, however, may occasionally be used to treat ovarian cancer under specific conditions.

1. Hormone therapy for tumors that have hormone receptors: Some cancers of the ovary have cells that have estrogen or progesterone receptors. In these situations, hormonal therapies like tamoxifen or aromatase inhibitors might be used to block these hormones' effects, which can aid in slowed tumor growth.

2. Maintenance therapy: Hormonal therapies, used after initial treatment with surgery and chemotherapy, may be used to stop or postpone the return of cancer. Oral contraceptives or aromatase inhibitors are just two examples of drugs that could be used in this situation.

3. Palliative care: Hormonal therapies may be used to help control symptoms and enhance the patient's quality of life in cases where ovarian cancer has spread to other body regions and is not responding to conventional treatments.

It is significant to remember that the efficacy of hormonal therapies for ovarian cancer varies depending on the patient and the unique features of the tumor. The oncologist will decide whether to use hormonal therapy and which medications to use based on a number of variables, including the cancer's stage, whether or not the tumor cells have hormone receptors, and the patient's general health.

CHAPTER 7

ADVANCED AND RECURRENT OVARIAN CANCER MANAGEMENT

7.1 Debulking Surgery

A surgical procedure frequently used in the management of ovarian cancer is debulking surgery, also referred to as cytoreductive surgery. It entails removing as much of the tumor as is feasible with the intention of lowering the tumor burden and enhancing the efficacy of subsequent therapies, such as chemotherapy.

When the cancer has returned or spread to other areas after initial treatment in the case of recurrent ovarian cancer, debulking surgery may be taken into consideration. The location and size of the recurrent tumor, the patient's general health, and their prior medical history all play a role in whether or not debulking surgery should be performed.

As well as any involved organs or tissues that are impacted by the cancer, the surgeon aims to remove all visible tumor masses during the procedure. The location and growth of the tumor will affect the surgery's scope. The removal of the uterus, nearby lymph nodes, ovaries, fallopian tubes, and other affected abdominal organs may be necessary in some circumstances.

In the management of recurrent ovarian cancer, debulking surgery has a variety of uses. It could aid in reducing pressure or pain brought on by tumor symptoms. The effectiveness of subsequent chemotherapy or other treatments can also be improved by debulking surgery because it lessens the burden of the tumor. The objective is to enhance the patient's quality of life and possibly extend survival.

It's crucial to keep in mind that debulking surgery is frequently carried out by a qualified gynecologic oncologist with experience performing ovarian cancer surgery. Debulking surgery should only be chosen after consulting with a medical staff that specializes in treating ovarian cancer and taking the patient's preferences and unique circumstances into account.

7.2 Continued Therapy

Following a first round of chemotherapy or other primary treatments, maintenance therapy for recurrent ovarian cancer typically entails ongoing care. The purpose of maintenance therapy is to increase overall survival rates and extend the time that the disease is under control or remission. The particular choice of maintenance therapy is based on a number of variables, including the circumstances unique to the patient, prior treatments received, and the characteristics of the cancer.

Common maintenance treatments for ovarian cancer recurrence include:

1. PARP Inhibitors: In ovarian cancer patients who responded to platinum-based chemotherapy, poly (ADP-ribose) polymerase (PARP) inhibitors like olaparib, niraparib, and rucaparib have demonstrated efficacy. The PARP enzyme, which is involved in DNA repair, is inhibited by these medications. By preventing PARP from functioning, cancer cells are unable to fix DNA damage and ultimately perish.

2. Bevacizumab: This targeted therapy prevents vascular endothelial growth factor (VEGF), a protein essential for angiogenesis (the growth of new blood vessels. Bevacizumab helps to restrict the blood supply to tumors, thereby limiting their growth, by blocking VEGF. As a maintenance therapy for recurrent ovarian cancer, it is frequently combined with chemotherapy.

3. Immunotherapy: Immune checkpoint inhibitors, like pembrolizumab and nivolumab, have shown promise in treating ovarian cancer patients who have tumors with particular genetic mutations, like DNA mismatch repair deficiency (dMMR) or high microsatellite instability (MSI-H). These medications support the body's immune system in identifying and combating cancer cells.

4. Hormone Therapy: Drugs used in hormone therapy, such as tamoxifen or aromatase inhibitors, may be used as maintenance therapy in cases where the ovarian cancer is hormone receptor positive. These medications inhibit estrogen's effects on cancer cells, which inhibits the growth of cancer cells.

It's crucial to remember that the decision regarding maintenance therapy should be made in consultation with a medical oncologist with experience treating ovarian cancer. To choose the most appropriate maintenance therapy, they will take into account a number of variables, such as the patient's general health, prior treatments, and the unique features of the recurrent cancer. Approach

7.3 Salvage Therapies

Salvage therapies are medical procedures used after the cancer has spread or returned after initial treatment. Symptom relief, disease management, and increased survival are the goals of salvage therapies. Here are a few typical salvage therapies for ovarian cancer that have returned:

1. Chemotherapy: Various chemotherapy medications or mixtures may be used to treat recurrent ovarian cancer. Platinum-based medications like cisplatin and carboplatin are frequently combined with other medications like paclitaxel or docetaxel. Chemotherapy can be administered intravenously or intraperitoneally (directly into the abdominal cavity) for greater effectiveness.

2. Targeted therapies: These treatments concentrate on a particular molecular or genetic abnormality that exists in cancer cells. Olaparib, rucaparib, and niraparib, which are PARP inhibitors, are a few examples of targeted therapies used in recurrent ovarian cancer. These medications specifically target cancer cells with faulty DNA repair systems.

3. Immunotherapy: Immunotherapy works to make the immune system of the body more effective at identifying and eliminating cancer cells. For a subset of ovarian cancers that show elevated levels of particular biomarkers like PD-L1, immune checkpoint inhibitors like pembrolizumab or nivolumab may be used.

4. Hormonal therapy: If your ovarian cancer has returned and it has hormone receptor positivity, hormonal therapy may be an option for you. To block hormone receptors and stop the spread of cancer, doctors may prescribe medications like tamoxifen or aromatase inhibitors.

5. Angiogenesis inhibitors: Angiogenesis inhibitors are medicines that prevent the development of brand-new blood vessels, which are essential for the growth of tumors. Angiogenesis inhibitors like bevacizumab can be combined with chemotherapy to treat recurrent ovarian cancer.

6. Clinical trials: Taking part in clinical trials can give you access to cutting-edge therapies that are still being tested as well as novel treatments. For recurrent ovarian cancer, clinical trials frequently evaluate brand-new medications, drug combinations, or therapeutic modalities.

It is significant to note that the decision regarding salvage therapy is influenced by a number of variables, including the patient's general health, the nature of the cancer, any prior treatments, and personal preferences. A medical or gynecologic oncologist should be consulted before choosing a course of treatment because they can make tailored suggestions based on the patient's unique circumstances.

PALLIATIVE CARE

Recurrent ovarian cancer is a term used to describe cancer that has come back or advanced following initial therapy. With a serious illness like recurrent ovarian cancer, palliative care aims to enhance the quality of life for patients. Palliative care aims to manage pain, relieve symptoms, and offer psychological and emotional support.

The following palliative care components may be taken into account for ovarian cancer that has returned:

1. Effective pain management is achieved through close patient collaboration with palliative care teams. To reduce pain and discomfort, they may combine medicine, physical therapy, and other methods.

2. Control Of Symptoms: Palliative care can address a number of symptoms related to recurrent ovarian cancer, including nausea, exhaustion, shortness of breath, and appetite loss. Enhancing comfort and general wellbeing is the main goal.

3. Support on an emotional and psychological level: Having recurrent ovarian cancer can be emotionally taxing. Social workers, counselors, or psychologists are frequently included on palliative care teams. They offer resources for coping with the emotional effects of the illness as well as emotional support and counseling.

4. Facilitating discussions between patients, their families, and healthcare professionals about treatment options, care objectives, and end-of-life planning is one of the main responsibilities of palliative care professionals. The wishes and values of the

patients are to be respected, they hope to ensure.

5. Care coordination: To ensure seamless coordination, palliative care teams collaborate with other healthcare professionals involved in the patient's care. They could support communication between specialists, assist with care transitions, and offer knowledge and instruction about the resources that are out there.

Depending on the needs and objectives of the patient, palliative care may be given in addition to curative therapies or as the main focus of treatment. Consult with medical experts, such as oncologists or palliative care specialists, who can offer individualized advice and support based on the particular circumstances if you or someone you know is dealing with recurrent ovarian cancer.

CHAPTER 8

SUPPORTIVE CARE AND QUALITY OF LIFE

Symptom management

It usually takes a multifaceted strategy that combines medical interventions, supportive care, and lifestyle changes to manage the symptoms of ovarian cancer. To create a personalized strategy for symptom management, it's critical to collaborate closely with a medical team that includes oncologists, nurses, and palliative care experts. To treat the signs of ovarian cancer, try some of the following methods:

- **Pain management**: Since pain is a frequent symptom of ovarian cancer, it can be treated with a variety of drugs, including nonsteroidal anti-inflammatory drugs (NSAIDs), opioids, and adjuvant analgesics. The best method of pain management will be chosen for you by your healthcare provider.

- **Vomiting and nauseousness**: Chemotherapy and other cancer treatments can make patients feel sick to their stomachs. To treat these symptoms, a doctor might prescribe antiemetic drugs like metoclopramide or ondansetron. Eating little and often can help, as can staying away from smelly or fatty foods that can be triggers.

- **Management of fatigue:** An ovarian cancer patient's tendency to feel tired is a common symptom. It is important to conserve energy, prioritize rest . It can be easier to manage fatigue if you mix up your activity with restful intervals. In order to maintain strength and energy levels, your healthcare team may also suggest gentle exercises or physical therapy.

- **Bowel and bladder problems:** Ovarian cancer can occasionally impair bowel and bladder function, resulting in signs and symptoms like constipation, diarrhea, or urinary issues. It is possible to control bowel movements with dietary changes like increasing fiber intake or drinking plenty of water. It may be necessary to prescribe medications like antidiarrheals or stool softeners. Referrals to experts like gastroenterologists or urologists may be required in certain circumstances.

- Support on an emotional level: Living with ovarian cancer can be difficult on an emotional level. In order to manage stress, anxiety, and depression, it can be helpful to seek support from close friends and family, join support groups, or seek professional counseling. It's possible that your medical staff will be able to suggest local resources for support services.

Support for proper nutrition is essential during the treatment of ovarian cancer. Any particular dietary needs or difficulties can be addressed with the aid of a registered dietitian when creating a personalized nutrition plan. They can also offer advice on how to handle changes in appetite, weight loss, or nutritional deficiencies.

- Interventions tailored to a particular symptom: Additional interventions may be required depending on the symptoms being experienced. Your medical team might use paracentesis to drain fluid, for instance, if ascites—an accumulation of fluid in the abdomen—occurs. Anticoagulant drugs may be prescribed to treat thrombosis (blood clots) in order to stop the formation of new clots.

Keep in mind that symptom management needs to be customized to your unique needs and preferences. Effective management requires open communication between you and your healthcare team about your symptoms and any new or escalating problems.

Support For Emotional And psychological Health In Regard To Fertility Preservation

For women with ovarian cancer, fertility preservation is crucial because some treatment options, like chemotherapy and radiation therapy, can negatively affect fertility. In order to successfully complete the fertility preservation process and manage the emotional difficulties brought on by ovarian cancer, women need support on a psychological and emotional level.

The following are a few techniques for offering psychological and emotional support:

1. Counseling and therapy: Women who have been diagnosed with ovarian cancer can gain from private counseling or therapy sessions with a psychologist or other mental health expert who specializes in cancer-related issues. Women can freely express their feelings, fears, and concerns during these sessions about preserving their fertility and the effects of the illness on their general wellbeing. Women can learn coping mechanisms and explore different stress-reduction techniques through counseling.

2. Support Groups: A support group specifically for ovarian cancer patients can be a huge help. It promotes a sense of community and understanding to interact with people who are experiencing comparable things. The chance to share experiences, learn new things, and get emotional support is provided by support groups. Additionally, they can connect women with resources and subject-matter experts, and they can offer information on options for fertility preservation.

3. Education and Information: It's crucial to make sure that women have access to accurate and thorough information about the various fertility preservation options. The various fertility preservation techniques that are available, their success rates, and any potential risks or side effects can all be explained by healthcare professionals in educational materials, brochures, and websites. Knowing this information empowers women to decide on their fertility in an informed manner and lessens anxiety and uncertainty.

4. Working with a Fertility Specialist: In order to achieve the best fertility preservation results, it is essential that the oncology team works closely with a fertility specialist. On methods for preserving fertility, such as egg freezing or embryo cryopreservation, in detail, consult a fertility specialist. Additionally, they can explain to women the timing of fertility preservation procedures in relation to cancer treatment and give them information on the potential effects of various treatment options on fertility.

5. Integrative therapies: Alternative methods, including meditation, yoga, and mindfulness exercises, can help lessen stress, anxiety, and depression related to ovarian cancer and fertility preservation. Integrative therapies may be provided in addition to traditional treatments to promote emotional resiliency and overall health.

It's crucial to tailor the support given because ovarian cancer patients' emotional and psychological needs differ from one another. Women can be given comprehensive care that addresses their physical, emotional, and fertility-related concerns by using a multidisciplinary approach involving oncologists, fertility experts, psychologists, and other medical professionals.

REHABILITATION AND SURVIVORSHIP NUTRITIONAL TIPS

Nutritional counseling is a crucial part of recovery and survival for ovarian cancer patients. A balanced diet can promote overall health, assist in coping with treatment side effects, and lower the likelihood of cancer recurrence. The following are some important nutritional factors for recovery and survivorship in ovarian cancer:

Consume a variety of foods from all food groups, such as fruits, vegetables, whole grains, lean proteins, and healthy fats. This is what is meant by eating a balanced diet. This offers necessary nutrients and promotes general health.

Increase your intake of fruits and vegetables because they are a good source of vitamins, minerals, antioxidants, and dietary fiber. For optimal health and to support immune function, aim for a minimum of five servings per day.

Select Whole Grains: Choose whole grains like oats, quinoa, oat bran, and whole wheat. Compared to refined grains, they offer more fiber, vitamins, and minerals, which helps to maintain bowel regularity and encourages satiety.

Lean sources of protein, such as poultry, fish, beans, and tofu, should be a part of your diet. Protein is crucial for immune system health, muscle mass preservation, and tissue repair.

Healthy Fats: Opt for sources of healthy fats like salmon, avocados, nuts, seeds, and olive oil. These fats support heart health and offer essential omega-3 fatty acids.

Drink plenty of water all day long to stay hydrated and support your body's general functions. Limit alcohol and sweet drinks.

Manage Digestive Issues: Following treatment or surgery, some ovarian cancer survivors may experience digestive problems. These symptoms may be controlled by eating small, frequent meals, drinking plenty of water, and avoiding greasy or spicy foods. For tailored advice, speak with a registered dietitian.

Describe Side Effects: Some ovarian cancer treatments, like chemotherapy, can have side effects like nausea, vomiting, or changes in taste. Develop management plans for these problems if you experience them by working with a healthcare team that includes a registered dietitian. This might entail eating more frequently and in smaller portions, experimenting with various flavors and textures, or adjusting the timing of meals and medication.

Maintain a Healthy Weight: Maintaining a healthy weight is good for your overall health and lowers your chance of getting cancer again. If necessary, create a specialized weight-management plan in collaboration with a registered dietitian.

Seek Professional Advice: Each person is unique, and dietary requirements can change depending on their personal preferences, medical conditions, and treatments. A registered dietitian with expertise in oncology should be consulted in order to receive individualized nutritional advice catered to your unique requirements.

Keep in mind that a thorough rehabilitation and survivorship plan for ovarian cancer includes more than just nutrition. Working closely with your medical team is crucial if you want to take care of all facets of your physical and psychological well-being.

CHAPTER 9

CLINICAL TRIALS AND THE FUTURE

Clinical Trials' Vitality

Our understanding of ovarian cancer is constantly evolving, and clinical trials are essential to improving patient outcomes. Here are some of the main arguments in favor of clinical trials for ovarian cancer:

1. Evaluating new treatments: Clinical trials examine the efficacy and safety of novel drugs, therapies, surgical procedures, and combinations of already-effective treatments. These studies are crucial for locating potential innovations that might improve the prognosis of ovarian cancer patients.

2. Improving the standard of care: Clinical trials contribute to establishing the current ovarian cancer standard of care. Researchers can determine whether a new treatment is more efficient, safer, or has fewer side effects by comparing it to the current standard of care. This information aids in the improvement of treatment protocols and the general standard of patient care.

3. Personalized medicine: Clinical trials shed light on ovarian cancer's genetic and molecular characteristics. This information aids in the identification of particular disease subtypes and guides the creation of focused treatments. Clinical trials enable scientists to test these personalized therapies on patients whose tumors have particular genetic mutations, enabling more specialized and efficient treatment approaches.

4. Early detection and prevention: Clinical trials concentrate on creating and assessing screening tools for ovarian cancer early detection. Research is currently being done to find efficient screening techniques and tools that can catch the disease in its earliest stages because early diagnosis can significantly increase survival rates. Trials focusing on preventive interventions, such as drugs or lifestyle changes, also aid in figuring out how to lower the risk of developing ovarian cancer.

5. Patient access to cutting-edge therapies: Enrolling in a clinical trial gives qualified patients access to innovative therapies that may not yet be widely accessible. Patients now have the chance to benefit from potential therapeutic advantages that might enhance their prognosis. Additionally, comprehensive medical care and monitoring are frequently offered as part of clinical trials, guaranteeing that participants receive the best possible care throughout the trial.

6. Increasing our understanding of science: Clinical trials produce insightful information that advances our understanding of ovarian cancer. This knowledge aids in the discovery of biomarkers, the development of new diagnostic techniques, and the improvement of therapeutic approaches. Clinical trial findings encourage ongoing improvements in ovarian cancer research and treatment, which benefits not only current patients but also future generations.

In conclusion, clinical trials are crucial for advancing our comprehension of ovarian cancer, creating novel therapeutic approaches, enhancing patient care, and ultimately aiming for better outcomes and elevated survival rates. Being involved in clinical trials is essential because it gives patients more control over their health, advances knowledge, and may lead to more individualized and effective treatment options.

PROMISING RESEARCH FIELDS

With numerous subtypes and difficult treatment options, ovarian cancer is a complicated disease. Researchers have been looking into a number of promising areas for improving the knowledge, diagnosis, and care of ovarian cancer over the years. The following are some ovarian cancer research areas that show promise:

The development of efficient screening techniques and biomarkers for early detection is essential for enhancing the prognosis for ovarian cancer. To detect ovarian cancer in its earliest stages, when treatment is most effective, researchers are investigating the use of blood tests, imaging methods, and genetic markers.

Personalized medicine: Ovarian cancer is a heterogeneous disease, which means that each person's experience with it is unique. In order to pinpoint specific molecular targets and subtypes of ovarian tumors, researchers are examining the genomic and molecular characteristics of these tumors. The outcomes for patients as a whole can be improved by customizing treatment plans.

Immunotherapy has recently transformed the way that cancer is treated. The immune system's capacity to identify and target ovarian cancer cells is being improved, according to researchers. For ovarian cancer, this includes the creation of immune checkpoint inhibitors, chimeric antigen receptor (CAR) T-cell therapy, and cancer vaccines to elicit immune responses.

Targeted therapies: Targeted therapies work to block particular molecules or signaling routes that contribute to the development of ovarian cancer. In order to create specific drugs that can target ovarian cancer cells only and leave healthy cells unharmed, researchers are identifying genetic mutations and molecular abnormalities in ovarian cancer cells. In comparison to conventional chemotherapy, these targeted therapies can enhance treatment effectiveness and minimize side effects.

Poly (ADP-ribose) polymerase (PARP) inhibitors have shown promise in the treatment of ovarian cancers caused by flaws in DNA repair mechanisms, such as those connected to BRCA gene mutations. The effectiveness of PARP inhibitors in various patient populations is currently being investigated, and combination therapies are being looked into to improve treatment outcomes.

Machine learning and Artificial Intelligence: A new area of ovarian cancer research is the use of machine learning (ML) and artificial intelligence (AI) to analyze large datasets and medical images. By predicting treatment outcomes, improving early detection, and creating individualized treatment plans based on unique patient characteristics, researchers are using these techniques.

Drug repurposing is the process of looking into the potential of using currently available medications for brand-new indications. The effectiveness of medications approved for other diseases against ovarian cancer is a topic of research. This strategy may speed up the creation of new treatments while also possibly lowering costs.

Quality of life and supportive care: Ovarian cancer and its treatments can have a big impact on patients' quality of life. In order to control treatment side effects, enhance emotional wellbeing, and increase survivability, researchers are concentrating on developing supportive care interventions.

It's crucial to keep in mind that even though these research areas have promise, putting them into clinical use and improving patient outcomes call for careful examination, clinical trials, and regulatory approval.

PERSONALIZED MEDICINE AND PRECISION ONCOLOGY

Precision oncology and personalized medicine are two interrelated paradigm shifts that have transformed the field of treating cancer, including ovarian cancer.

Personalizing medical decisions and interventions for each patient based on their particular traits, such as their genetic make-up, lifestyle choices, and environmental exposures, is a key component of personalized medicine. This method takes into account the fact that every patient is unique and that a treatment plan that is successful for one patient might not be for another.

Contrarily, precision oncology specializes in the treatment of cancer and uses cutting-edge technologies to examine the molecular makeup of a patient's tumor. Doctors can choose targeted therapies that are more likely to be successful by comprehending the genetic mutations and other changes driving the cancer's growth.

In the case of ovarian cancer, precision oncology and personalized medicine have significantly improved patient outcomes. Some examples of how these techniques have been used are as follows:

To identify specific mutations or alterations in a patient's tumor DNA, genetic testing is the first step in personalized medicine. Analysis of genes like BRCA1 and BRCA2, which are linked to an increased risk of developing ovarian and breast cancers, may be part of ovarian cancer testing. Genetic testing can support informed treatment choices and help identify patients who might gain from clinical trials or targeted therapies.

2. Targeted Therapies: Precision oncology searches for targeted treatments that can ostensibly block the signaling molecules or pathways that are responsible for tumor growth. Targeted treatments for ovarian cancer, like poly(ADP-ribose) polymerase (PARP) inhibitors, have shown promise, especially in patients with BRCA mutations. These medications improve treatment outcomes because they take advantage of the unique weaknesses present in cancer cells with these mutations.

3. Immunotherapy: The creation of immunotherapies is another area of precision oncology research in ovarian cancer. Immunotherapies encourage the body's defenses to identify and target cancer cells. In order to improve the immune response against ovarian cancer cells, researchers are looking into a variety of immunotherapy techniques, such as immune checkpoint inhibitors, adoptive cell transfer, and cancer vaccines.

4. Prognostic and Predictive Biomarkers: Precision oncology and personalized medicine look for biomarkers that can foretell a patient's response to a particular course of treatment and direct the course of that treatment. For instance, specific biomarkers could be used to identify which patients are more likely to benefit from targeted or chemotherapy treatments. Using this knowledge can help prevent ineffective treatments and lessen unneeded side effects.

5. Clinical Trials: Precision oncology and personalized medicine have made it easier to create clinical trials that focus on particular molecular alterations in ovarian cancer. Researchers can assess a subset of patients who are more likely to benefit from new therapies by choosing patients based on their tumor profiles. The likelihood of finding novel treatments suited to patients' specific needs rises as a result of this strategy.

By offering targeted therapies, improving patient selection for clinical trials, and optimizing treatment decisions based on individual characteristics, personalized medicine and precision oncology have, overall, changed the landscape of ovarian cancer treatment. These methods show great promise for future developments in the field, which will improve patient outcomes and quality of life.

Innovative Treatment Methods

Although ovarian cancer is a difficult condition to treat, several cutting-edge strategies have been created recently. Some of the significant developments:

Poly (ADP-ribose) polymerase (PARP) inhibitors have demonstrated efficacy in the management of ovarian cancer, particularly in those with BRCA gene mutations. These inhibitors prevent cancer cells from using their DNA repair mechanisms, which ultimately kills the cells. Advanced ovarian cancer has been approved for treatment with medications like Olaparib, Niraparib, and Rucaparib.

Immunotherapy: A small number of ovarian cancer patients have shown some benefit from immune checkpoint inhibitors like Pembrolizumab and Nivolumab. By inhibiting the proteins that suppress immune responses, these medications trigger the body's immune system to attack cancer cells. To improve treatment effectiveness, combination therapies are also being investigated. One such combination is immune checkpoint inhibitors and PARP inhibitors.

Targeted Therapies: Targeted therapies work to block particular molecules that contribute to the development and spread of cancer. For example, the angiogenesis inhibitor bevacizumab, which targets the vascular endothelial growth factor (VEGF), is combined with chemotherapy for advanced ovarian cancer. Inhibitors of the HER2/neu pathway, mTOR pathway, and other signaling pathways are among the other targeted treatments being researched.

Antibody-Drug Conjugates (ADCs): ADCs are a new class of medications that combine the cytotoxicity of chemotherapy with the specialized properties of monoclonal antibodies. The harm to healthy tissues is reduced because these medications deliver chemotherapy directly to cancer cells. ADCs like Trastuzumab emtansine (T-DM1) and Mirvetuximab soravtansine have shown promise in ovarian cancer clinical trials.

Precision Medicine: The development of genomic profiling and molecular testing has aided the use of precision medicine techniques in the treatment of ovarian cancer. Treatment options can be influenced by determining the precise genetic mutations and alterations present in tumors. This includes identifying patients who might benefit from immunotherapy or targeted therapies based on their molecular profiles.

Specifically when the disease has spread to the peritoneal cavity, advanced ovarian cancer patients may benefit from hyperthermic intraperitoneal chemotherapy

(HIPEC). After removing visible tumors surgically, heated chemotherapy is then administered directly into the abdominal cavity. The chemotherapy works more efficiently and specifically on remaining cancer cells at the higher temperature.

The efficacy and safety of each of these cutting-edge treatment modalities may differ depending on the unique patient characteristics, despite the fact that they all appear to have promise. A qualified oncologist should be consulted before choosing a course of treatment so they can take each patient's unique situation into account.

CONCLUSION

ovarian cancer remains a significant and formidable health challenge for women worldwide. Its insidious nature, often presenting with subtle or vague symptoms in its early stages, makes early detection and intervention a critical factor in improving survival rates and patient outcomes. Despite advancements in research and medical technology, there is still much work to be done in understanding the complex biology and risk factors associated with this disease.

The development of targeted therapies and immunotherapies shows promise in providing more effective treatment options with fewer side effects. However, these treatments are still evolving, and continued research is essential to optimize their potential.

Awareness campaigns and education about the signs and risk factors of ovarian cancer are crucial in encouraging early detection and empowering women to take charge of their health. Regular screenings and genetic testing for high-risk individuals can play a significant role in identifying the disease at its earliest stages.

Collaboration among researchers, clinicians, and advocacy groups is vital in advancing ovarian cancer research and patient care. Increased funding and support for research initiatives are necessary to unravel the complexities of this disease and develop innovative approaches for prevention, diagnosis, and treatment.

Ultimately, the fight against ovarian cancer requires a multi-faceted approach, from empowering individuals with knowledge and awareness to advancing scientific discoveries and healthcare infrastructure. By combining efforts on all fronts, we can strive towards a future where ovarian cancer is more effectively managed and one day, even conquered.

Dear Esteemed Customers,

Permit us to express our gratitude for your decision to read our book at this time.We sincerely appreciate your unwavering support and insightful criticism. As we strive to consistently improve our work and provide thought-provoking content, we sincerely appreciate your cooperation in the form of a candid evaluation.

Your reviews not only give us authors crucial information, but they also guide prospective readers in making informed decisions. We sincerely appreciate your feedback, regardless of how much you enjoy the book or how strongly you believe that there are some things that could have been handled more expertly. Your feedback encourages us to keep writing books that connect with you.

Please take a moment to post your Amazon review.Your opinions will have a big impact on our book's marketing and its potential audience.

Remember that your review doesn't have to be lengthy or in-depth. It will be very helpful to simply state your personal beliefs, draw attention to passages that spoke to you, or highlight noteworthy details.

We sincerely value your assistance and participation.
we can't wait to read your comments.

APPENDIX: GLOSSARY OF TERMS

Here's a glossary of Terms related to ovarian cancer:

1. Ovarian Cancer: A type of cancer that originates in the ovaries, which are the female reproductive organs responsible for producing eggs and hormones.

2. Tumor: An abnormal growth or mass of cells. In the case of ovarian cancer, it refers to the abnormal growth of cells in the ovaries.

3. Benign: Non-cancerous. A benign tumor does not spread to other parts of the body and is usually not life-threatening.

4. Malignant: Cancerous. A malignant tumor has the potential to invade nearby tissues and spread to other parts of the body, leading to serious health complications.

5. Metastasis: The spread of cancer from its original site to other parts of the body. In ovarian cancer, metastasis may occur when cancer cells from the ovaries invade nearby organs or travel through the bloodstream or lymphatic system to form tumors in distant organs.

6. Epithelial Ovarian Cancer (EOC): The most common type of ovarian cancer, accounting for about 90% of cases. It originates in the cells that line the surface of the ovaries.

7. Germ Cell Tumor: A type of ovarian cancer that develops from the cells that produce eggs. Germ cell tumors are relatively rare and often occur in younger women.

8. Stromal Tumor: A type of ovarian cancer that develops in the cells that produce female hormones. Stromal tumors are less common than epithelial ovarian cancer and usually have a better prognosis.

9. BRCA1 and BRCA2: Genes that produce proteins that help suppress the growth of tumors. Mutations in these genes increase the risk of developing ovarian and breast cancer.

10. Risk Factors: Conditions or factors that increase the likelihood of developing a disease. In the case of ovarian cancer, risk factors include age, family history of ovarian or breast cancer, certain gene mutations, personal history of breast or colorectal cancer, and certain reproductive factors.

11. Screening: The process of testing individuals who are at risk of a particular disease to detect it at an early stage. Ovarian cancer screening typically involves a combination of pelvic examinations, transvaginal ultrasound, and blood tests.

12. CA-125: A protein that is often elevated in the blood of women with ovarian cancer. CA-125 blood test is commonly used to monitor ovarian cancer or detect its recurrence, but it is not specific to ovarian cancer and can be elevated in other conditions.

13. Chemotherapy: The administration of medications to treat or prevent the growth and division of cancer cells. Chemotherapy is a frequent form of treatment for ovarian cancer and can be given intravenously or intraperitoneally.

14. Radiation therapy: The use of powerful radiation to destroy cancer cells or reduce tumors. Although it is less frequently used, radiation therapy may be suggested in some cases for the treatment of ovarian cancer.

15. Surgery: The primary treatment for ovarian cancer involves the surgical removal of the tumor and, in some cases, the ovaries, fallopian tubes, uterus, and nearby lymph nodes. The extent of surgery depends on the stage and characteristics of the cancer.

16. Stage: A way of describing the extent and spread of cancer in the body. Ovarian cancer stages range from I to IV, with stage I being confined to the ovaries and stage IV indicating the cancer has spread to distant organs.

17. Prognosis: The likely outcome or course of a disease. The prognosis for ovarian cancer depends on various factors, including the stage at diagnosis, tumor grade, the age and general health of the patient, and response to treatment.

Made in United States
Troutdale, OR
09/06/2023

12697699R00086